THE VACCINATION TABOO

BY JAMES JOSEPH COOK

You can tell a lot about a society by what ordinary people talk about at parties and over the dinner table. You can tell a lot more by what people don't talk about.

Back in the mid-nineteenth century, Southern whites didn't chit-chat about the horrors of slavery, nor did Northern businessmen talk about the hellish lives of factory and mine laborers. Easterners didn't discuss the plight of immigrants in ghettos and Westerners kept quiet about the extermination of the natives.

Most of us, it seems, think today's America is different. Now we talk about anything and everything: same-sex marriage, global warming, March Madness, GMO labeling, the most recent episode of <u>Game of Thrones</u>, the glory or folly of the latest U.S. military adventure, the features of Iphone nth, the advance of ISIS, the xxx installment of the action-adventure flavor of the week, the starving children of India, what color underpants this politician or that celebrity wore when he or she posted a risqué selfie on Facebook, the latest dance or diet craze, etc., etc.

What we don't talk about, most of us, is vaccination.

Why is that?

Maybe it's because, as Frank Bruni of the New York Times put it in a tirade against anti-vaxxers ironically titled "The Vaccine Lunacy," "This subject has been studied and studied and studied, and it's abundantly clear that we're best served by vaccinating all of those children who can be, so that the ones who can't be — for medical reasons such as a compromised immune system — are protected." [http://www.nytimes.com/2015/02/01/opinion/sunday/frank-bruni-disneyland-measles-and-madness.html]

Notice, he doesn't say that he's studied the subject of vaccination, just that it's been studied, implying that the experts who have studied it have all arrived at the same conclusion. So for a rational person further discussion is crazy and we should all just leave it at that.

Some crazy people, who in a different age would have been the ones called rational, can't leave it at that. They actually have the temerity to ask who are these experts and what have they actually found. They have the chutzpa not to care if the general public ridicules them as wing nuts, fear-mongers, and even criminals. For the sake of their own health and that of their children, they are stupid enough not to trust the powers that be and to investigate vaccines for themselves.

After all, stripped of all the emotional trappings, the issue is straightforward and simple: do vaccines really protect us from deadly infectious disease, or do they not? Are vaccines safe and effective, or are they dangerous and maybe even destructive? What does the actual science say?

Before getting into those issues, though, it's important to understand what a vaccine is. In simple terms, a vaccine is an antigen injected or ingested in order to stimulate an immune response. But just as with almost everything else in life, it's not nearly that simple.

The whole point of any vaccine, according to medical orthodoxy, is to stimulate the immune system to form a ready-response team of antibodies in the bloodstream that can search out and destroy a targeted maleficent microbe. This response is elicited by fooling the immune system into thinking it's under attack by that microbe. In other words, vaccination is a drill. After the drill these specialized antibodies (all antibodies are specialized) will hang around so they can leap into action if and when the real live bad microbe they are designed to destroy does invade. This is the meaning of "vaccine-induced immunity."

So vaccines are just different ways to sound a false alarm. The National Institute of Allergies and Infectious Diseases (NIAID), part of the National Institutes of Health (NIH), lists seven types of vaccines, the last two of which are still in the experimental stage:

1. Live attenuated vaccine, which uses a microbe that's been brought to the verge of death so it can't do any real harm.

2. Inactivated vaccine, which uses a killed or inactivated microbe.

3. Subunit vaccine, which uses a piece of a microbe.

4. Toxoid vaccine, which employs a "detoxified" toxin secreted by a microbe.

5. Conjugated vaccine, for babies whose inexperienced immune systems can't yet recognize the targeted pathogen as a bad guy, so it's coupled with a mean-faced antigen wearing a black hat.

6. DNA vaccine, which uses only the DNA of the targeted microbe. This type is touted as taking the technology to a whole new level, because presumably foreign DNA injected into the bloodstream can scare the bejesus out of the immune system without doing as much real harm as it could if it were inside its original microbe.

7. Recombinant vector vaccine, in which the aforementioned isolated DNA does have a microbial carrier, but only as a delivery system.

But all this tech talk shouldn't obscure the fact that different types of vaccines are just different ways the biotechnicians can put on a play for the immune system: a horror show that has to be realistic enough to scare the immune system into thinking the organism is under lethal attack, but not so realistic as to do any actual physiological damage. Funny, with all the undisputed scientific evidence that stress is an etiological factor in many diseases, you might think that fright alone would cause harm, especially to a little baby. But Dr. Paul Offit, the seemingly omnipresent establishment mouthpiece (who, purely parenthetically and by the way, has made tens if not hundreds of millions of dollars from the patenting and sale of vaccines that he himself, as a member of the CDC Advisory Board, voted onto the schedule) assures us that a baby can well tolerate the administering of 10,000 (yes, the four zeros are intentional) vaccine doses in one day. Did he try this on himself?

[http://vactruth.com/2015/04/23/baby-dies-after-13-vaccines/?utm_source=The+Vaccine+Truth+Ne

wsletter&utm_campaign=0a78af229e-
04_23_2015_bently&utm_medium=email&utm_
term=0_ce7860ee83-0a78af229e-408394085]

Vaccine antigens cannot be patented, and therefore vaccines cannot be profitable, unless those antigens are in some way synthetic and not found in nature. (Dr. Frankenstein, anyone?) Yet they are supposed to produce antibodies against a microbe that is found in nature, and antibodies are highly specific. Okay.

In any case, vaccine antigens are microbes, or pieces thereof, and therefore require an organic habitat in which to survive and thrive. Bacterial antigens are propagated in petri dishes, but viruses are grown in organic tissue from monkey kidneys, dog kidneys, mouse brains, chicken embryos, pig gelatin, fetal cow blood, diploid cells from aborted human fetuses, armyworms, etc. Of course, this organic tissue is teeming with who knows how many potential contaminants, and little effort is made to filter the noxious brews. Testing for every possible known contaminant would be prohibitively costly, and the unknown contaminants can't be tested for because, well, they're unknown. But, presumably, the methods used to attenuate or inactivate the antigen will also disable or kill all the other pathogens, known or unknown.

Or maybe not. Viruses in particular are tricky

critters. Like possums, they can play dead. They bridge the gap between the animate and the inanimate, and so partake of the qualities of both. Think of a life form that can turn to stone when threatened and reanimate itself when the threat has passed. Likewise, microbes of whatever sort have the evolutionary edge of multiplying far more rapidly than larger life forms. This enables them to adapt to harsh conditions created by the heat or poisons biotechnicians employ to kill them. How, one might wonder, can the experts be so certain that inactivated, much less attenuated microbes, as well as any parts thereof, aren't just taking a nap until they are transported, courtesy of your doctor's trusty hypodermic needle, into the land of milk and honey where they can reactivate, regroup, infiltrate and conquer, all before anyone is the wiser?

Besides antigens, vaccines contain a variety of toxic substances that serve as adjuvants and preservatives. An adjuvant strengthens the immune response, so by definition it must be toxic. Adjuvants are needed because the attenuated or inactivated antigen may not stimulate a strong enough immune response. Yes, that's right. They attenuate or inactivate the antigen so it won't do any real harm. But then the adaptive immune system may recognize the deception and not produce the desired antibodies, so they add a toxic adjuvant so the immune system will realize the antigen is not just an idle threat – like discovering that your bad-boy date is the sweetest guy in the world, but then getting raped by his tag-along brother. Got that?

A preservative kills contaminants and preserves the inactivated antigen, so it is also by definition toxic.

Since the 1920s aluminum has been the adjuvant of choice. Until recently, mercury was the most common preservative, and it's still used in the injected flu vaccine and in "trace amounts" in others. But because of the outcry against mercury in recent years, now aluminum often does double duty as both adjuvant and preservative. Never mind that aluminum is nearly as deadly a neurotoxin as mercury and so crosses the blood-brain barrier with equal ease. Never mind that the blood-brain barrier isn't even fully developed until adolescence. The NIAID, the Centers for Disease Control (CDC) and a host of other authorities, including Dr. Offit, assure us that aluminum is abundant in nature and humans are constantly ingesting it. What they fail to mention, though Dr. Suzanne Humphries does, is that your body absorbs only 1-2% of the aluminum (or mercury, for that matter) that may be in your food and drink, but 100% of what's injected into you.

[http://articles.mercola.com/sites/articles/archive/2015/03/31/aluminum-vaccines.aspx]

And don't worry about the fact that the kind of aluminum in vaccines is much more toxic than that found naturally in the environment, especially when injected into the muscles rather than directly into the bloodstream, as it is with some vaccines in order to minimize the risk of inducing an allergy to peanuts because of the refined peanut oil often used as a coadjuvant. Yes, peanut oil, though it doesn't have to be listed in the ingredients because the FDA classifies it as GRAS (generally recognized as safe). Any connection with the sudden rise of deadly peanut allergies in the last few decades? [Dr. Tim O'Shea, Vaccination Is Not Immunization, 4th ed., 2015, pp. 84ff.: http://www.amazon.com/Vaccination-Not-Immunization-4th-Fourth-ebook/dp/B00UCO6BG6/ref=sr_1_1?s=books&ie=UTF8&qid=1451507991&sr=1-1&keywords=vaccination+is+not+immunization]

And then of course there are the "trace amounts" of formaldehyde, which is just as good at preserving vaccines as it is at preserving dead bodies, and also as effective in attenuating or inactivating targeted microbes as the FBI found it to be in killing wayward imbibers when that

government agency added it to alcohol during Prohibition.
[http://www.naturalnews.com/029029_Prohibition_poisoning.html] But of course in vaccines, unlike anywhere else, formaldehyde behaves like a perfect gentleman.

As you may be starting to realize, this vaccine horror show boasts a cast of villains that rivals anything Hollywood has produced, and with the development of nanotechnology they promise to get even scarier. Only, the monsters featured in this melodrama aren't make-believe. Just like in boot camp, that's live ammunition whizzing over our heads, or rather, racing through our blood streams. But even though vaccines sound like something out of a campy science-fiction novel, the real issue remains to be considered: Do they work?

The clear assumption of the vaccine establishment is that it is much smarter than both the human immune system and the microbes that attack it. The CDC admits that natural immunity is superior to vaccine-induced immunity except in one respect: it takes a while to develop, and if you wait around for it to kick in instead of getting vaccinated, you could well die in the meantime.
[http://www.cdc.gov/vaccines/pubs/parents-

guide/downloads/parents-guide-part3.pdf]
Prominent scientists, physicians, public health authorities, most politicians, and the average ordinary citizen all hail vaccination as one of the greatest medical inventions of all time. They repeatedly claim that vaccines have saved millions upon millions of lives. The CDC, the World Health Organization (WHO), your warm and fuzzy pediatrician, and those cute nurses on public health department web sites all assure us that vaccines are safe and effective. Dr. Offit even brought Jesus into the debate in a NY Times op-ed, "What Would Jesus Do About Measles?", saying that the Man from Nazareth loved children so much that, if he were around today, he would eliminate all exemptions based on philosophy or religious belief and support mandatory vaccination, no ifs, ands or buts. [http://www.nytimes.com/2015/02/10/opinion/what-would-jesus-do-about-measles.htm] Never mind that the CDC estimates that only 10% of vaccine injuries are actually reported, and others put the figure at 1-2%. [http://www.nvic.org/reportreaction.aspx] Never mind that the U.S. government set up a National Vaccine Injury Compensation Board (VICB) in 1986 when it so considerately relieved vaccine manufacturers of any legal liability for the damage a vaccine may cause, and that VICB has

had to pay out $124 million in legal fees and almost $3 billion to the lucky few with the grit, savvy and resources to out-shoot its top-gun lawyers. [http://www.infowars.com/the-us-government-has-paid-out-3-billion-to-vaccine-injured-americans-since-1989/] Never mind that all vaccines arrive at the doctor's office with inserts warning of possible side-effects ranging from mild fever and rashes to severe seizures, encephalopathy, coma, and anaphylactic shock – information most doctors choose not to share with their patients. [http://www.vaccinesafety.edu/package_inserts.htm]

Most people, even pediatricians when they're not talking to paying customers, are honest enough to admit that vaccines come with a trade-off: a statistically rare individual might have a serious adverse reaction, but it's all for the greater good. Vaccines, they aver, have saved many more people than they've hurt. That vaccines are effective is beyond scientific doubt.

You might think that numerous clinical studies have demonstrated that vaccines really do save lives, but in point of fact there are none, at least none recognized by the medical establishment. For allegedly ethical reasons, that establishment shies away from comparing vaccinated to unvaccinated populations.

Presumably, it's not right to even allow an unvaccinated population to exist. So are they lying?

Well, it depends on what you mean by lying. You see, "effective" and "protection" don't mean the same thing in vaccine-speak as they do in everyday life. If someone says that vaccines have been clinically proven to provide effective protection against disease, you would naturally assume that people who otherwise would have gotten said disease didn't because they were vaccinated. Vaccine proponents make such claims all the time, but these claims are based not on proof but the assumption that the vaccination-hypothesis is true. When they talk about proven effectiveness, they mean a given vaccine has been shown to elicit in most individuals tested the desired immune response. That's it. That's their "proof" of effectiveness.

And when it comes to protection, the claim for just about every vaccine at its inception was that it would bestow immunity for life. When that claim proved false, there developed the concepts of revaccination and vaccination-induced herd immunity. The immunity allegedly bestowed by vaccination would wear off, and so repeated vaccination was necessary. When even revaccinated people proved susceptible to the targeted disease, there came the admission that vaccination only worked in a portion of a given population; but if enough of that population were vaccinated, that would protect both the ones in whom it didn't work and the unvaccinated. This doctrine of vaccine-induced herd-immunity is the allegedly scientific rationale for universal mandatory vaccination.

I think Offit was right to bring Jesus into the vaccine conversation, because he gave the simplest and clearest definition of the scientific method ever: "By their fruits you shall know them" (Matthew 7:16). So, from a scientific as well as moral perspective, the fundamental question about vaccines is this: Are they so effective at supporting the human immune system that they're worth all the fuss and bother, all the possible side-effects and life-threatening reactions? If the few are to be sacrificed for the many, we better be damn sure that the sacrifice is not in vain. But since none of the vaccine-establishment players, government or corporate, is willing to fund a large-scale study comparing the health of the vaccinated to that of the unvaccinated, we seem to have come to a dead-end. Fortunately, at least for those of us who realize that the world did not begin when we were born, history provides the answer.

The most exhaustively researched, meticulously documented, and scientifically

grounded work on the history of vaccination is
Dissolving Illusions: Disease, Vaccines, and the
Forgotten History by Suzanne Humphries, MD
and Roman Bystrianyk
[http://www.amazon.com/Dissolving-Illusions-
Disease-Vaccines-
Forgotten/dp/1480216895/ref=sr_1_1?s=books&
ie=UTF8&qid=1430240536&sr=1-
1&keywords=dissolving+illusions+disease+vacc
ines+and+the+forgotten+history]. Dr.
Humphries gave up a successful 19-year career
as a nephrologist when three of her patients,
without her permission, were routinely
vaccinated upon admission to her hospital and
suffered a rapid deterioration of their condition
that resulted in one case in death. She decided to
find out if all she had been taught and routinely
accepted about vaccines was really true. Ten
years of research later the conclusion was
impossible to evade: Vaccines have done nothing
to stop the diseases for whose disappearance
they've been given the credit, and they have been
responsible for untold misery and death.

Consider Edward Jenner's invention, the
granddaddy of all vaccines, the smallpox
vaccine. Jenner was a lousy scientist who in
1796 launched his glorious career on the basis of
a milkmaid superstition and one dubious clinical
trial of a young boy, but he was also a brilliant

salesman who wheedled 30,000 pounds (millions in today's money) out of the British government to develop his vaccine. The politicians weren't scientists at all, but they saw how to buttress their careers as well as the power of government by mandating vaccination under the pretext of saving the world from smallpox. And most physicians, many of whom originally opposed vaccination, fell in line when they saw what it did for their incomes. Inconveniently, however, throughout the 19th century the worst smallpox epidemics struck wherever and whenever vaccination rates were the highest. And we're talking very high rates, since in most modernizing countries, East and West, as well as in those countries under European control like India, vaccination and revaccination were mandated and those mandates were enforced.

To give just a few examples from the many found in this book, by 1870 Prussia probably had the highest revaccination rate anywhere in the world. Nevertheless, when the worst smallpox epidemic of the century hit in 1871, nearly 60,000 died of smallpox. A few decades later Japan was even more heavily revaccinated, yet people died of smallpox at a higher rate than before mass vaccination.

On the other hand, in 1885 the people of Leicester, England rebelled against mandatory vaccination, threw out the local government that supported it and voted in a new government that favored freedom of choice. At the same time, they took measures to improve public nutrition, sanitation and hygiene, as well as to humanely quarantine anyone who came down with smallpox and their families. The incidence of smallpox dropped to a fourth of that in heavily vaccinated Birmingham and the mortality rate to one-tenth. All the establishment experts and pundits, including the editors of the major newspapers like the <u>New York Times</u> (Shades of Bruni and Offit!), predicted for Leicester apocalyptic doom. Smallpox disappeared from Leicester faster than anywhere else in Britain, and it never returned. It disappeared from Europe and America as mandatory vaccination laws were revoked, the rate of vaccination fell and dramatic improvements were made in (yes, you guessed it) public nutrition, sanitation and hygiene.

And so it went with all the infectious diseases for whose disappearance vaccines and antibiotics, the bread-and-butter drugs of the pharmaceutical industry, have been credited.

With such a damning historical critique out there in the world, you might think that the vaccine establishment would publish its own equally detailed history, just as firmly rooted in primary sources, to contest it. Of course the trolls, those Brown Shirts of the Internet, attack Dr. Humphries when opportunity arises. One finds the usual character assassination, as well as begging-the-question and technical sniping disguised as scientific debunking and refutation, most of it anonymous; but there's nothing nearly as comprehensive, cogent and convincing. And one has to wonder what Dr. Humphries had to gain from giving up a career as a stellar nephrologist in a major hospital in order to devote ten years of her life to formulating so elaborate a hoax. Who are the wing-nut conspiracy theorists here?

All the trollish nitpicking, plausible deniability and media propaganda cannot hide the truth that the world, and especially the United States, is fundamentally different since the resurrection of mass vaccination over half a century ago and its progressive multiplication from a few doses of a handful of vaccines to 49 doses of 14 vaccines by the time a child starts kindergarten and 64 doses of 16 vaccines by the time she finishes high school. Estimates of the current rate of childhood autism vary between one child in a hundred and one in fifty, but fifty years ago only one in 10,000 children developed autism. Heart disease, cancer and asthma were once largely confined to the old and weak, but now they are found in small children and infants at rates so high that the government is assisting hospitals in the development of an end-of-life-care program for babies. Rankings vary, but no one can deny that the infant-mortality rate in this country, which has steadily gone down in the last century, is now stagnating, going from one of the lowest to one of the highest in the developed world, if not the whole world [http://europepmc.org/abstract/med/19887034].

In his Vaccination Is Not Immunization [http://www.immunitionltd.com/book/vaccination-is-not-immunization.htm], which clearly details the horrific history vaccine by deadly vaccine, Dr. Tim O'Shea says that 53,000 infants die each year of terminal disease and 11,300 newborns die on the first day of life, 50% more than in all the other developed countries combined. The U.S. is the only country in the world to vaccinate an infant on the first day of life. Are we to believe that this is all coincidence? Americans are the most heavily vaccinated people in the world. If vaccines do what the authorities claim they do, shouldn't we be the healthiest?

For those who have a mind to inquire and eyes to see, there's plenty of other evidence out there that vaccination causes death and destruction and has done nothing to improve the collective health of the human race. With one voice, the medical establishment declares that the people who unearth and present this evidence can't possibly know what they're talking about because they aren't experts in the field of immunology. That's like the authorities of Galileo's day saying he knew nothing about astronomy because he denied that the heavenly spheres moved in perfect circles. Just as with the Catholic Church in the Middle Ages, anyone who challenges the vaccination dogma is ipso facto a charlatan, banned from the communion of the faithful and condemned as a wing-nut heretic. However, as with the movement of the planets, once you get past the orthodoxy's gobbledygook, the actual science relevant to vaccination is clear and understandable to anyone with an open mind.

Modern medicine, which considers itself the only valid and scientific form of medicine, is allopathy. The allopathic attitude, which permeates our culture, is nicely summed up by the top-shelf immunologist in <u>World War Z</u> shortly before he accidentally blows himself away and leaves Brad Pitt to fight the zombie epidemic on his own: "Mother Nature is a bitch." She and her killer microbes lie in wait for all of us unless we can outsmart her with our high-tech drugs. Medical technology alone can save us.

Vaccines are our primo weapons against the vicious microbes; but they only work if no gaps are left in the defenses, if everyone willy-nilly is vaccinated.

The two cutting-edge fields of research in contemporary biology and medicine are epigenetics and the study of the human microbiome. It is becoming increasingly clear that allopathy gets just about everything wrong when it comes to nature, health and life. Just as epigenetics shows that genes are like light switches, turned on and off by extra-genetic factors like environment and diet; so too does current microbiology reveal that germs are not the source of disease. We live in a teeming sea of microbes, many of which are essential to every one of our vital functions: digestion, respiration, waste elimination, neurological communication, and yes, protection from disease. We could not eat, think, breathe, detoxify or survive without millions and billions of viruses and bacteria helping us. These microbes make up our microbiome. Allopathy treats microbes as the enemy. If microbes are really our friends, where does that place allopathy?

The fundamental fallacy of vaccination, that herd-immunity can be artificially induced, stems from the failure to distinguish between the innate immune system and the adaptive immune system. It is the reduction of the complex and organic development of natural immunity to a specific response of the adaptive immune system.

Maleficent microbes aren't out there just waiting for a chance to invade and conquer. As Dave Yong, a science writer for National Geographic, put it, "'Healthy microbes can easily turn rogue. Those in our guts are undoubtedly helpful, but if they cross the lining of the intestine and enter our bloodstream, they can trigger a debilitating immune response. The same microbes can be beneficial allies or dangerous threats, all for the difference of a few millimeters." [http://www.nytimes.com/2014/11/02/opinion/sunday/there-is-no-healthy-microbiome.html In other words, infectious disease is a function of misplaced microbes.

The poliomyelitis virus, to take an example from Dissolving Illusions, was a benign member of the human gut flora (and, as far as anyone knows, still is) until at mid-20th century Americans fell in love with DDT, the terminator of evil germs, and sprayed it not only on their

lawns and gardens but food and bedding too. The
countries like India where "wild" polio (polio
not caused by the polio vaccine) still exists are
also today's primary producers and users of
DDT, a chemical now banned almost everywhere
else. Incidentally, in India as everywhere else,
the polio vaccine has done nothing but cause a
lot more murder and mayhem than polio itself.

What keeps microbes in their proper place in
the human microbiome? First of all, physical
barriers like the skin and the mucous membranes
that cover the digestive, urinary, reproductive,
and respiratory tracts. If an antigen, or foreign
protein, gets through these barriers, the innate
immune system kicks in with a wide range of
defensive weapons, mostly white blood cells and
supporting proteins. If an antigen happens to
pierce this second line of defense, then the
adaptive immune system comes into play, using
information transmitted from the innate immune
system to develop antibodies that specifically
target the invader and bring about its destruction.
Even if the invader doesn't make it through the
innate immune system's defenses, that system
still transmits intelligence that enables the entire

immune system to remember the invader and destroy it next time it crosses the body's borders. There are exceptions, like measles, which the innate immune system usually handles on its own; but generally, this is how natural, long-lasting immunity to specific pathogens develops.

However, perhaps martial metaphors are not the best way of characterizing the human immune system. Immunity might better be called "harmony." It is a characteristic not of this system or that, but of the organism as a whole. In a garden with healthy soil-structure, soil critters and ground-cover, weeds are not a problem. In a society founded on justice, compassion and creativity, crime is at a minimum. In an organism that is well nourished, well exercised, and exposed to plenty of sunlight and fresh air, disease finds no foothold.

Because it is maintained by thoroughly natural means, the innate immune system can never make pharmaceutical corporations tons of liability-free profits. Nevertheless, it is the foundation of all herd-immunity. In a society in harmony with nature, which means functioning according to the ecology of living beings, the weakest members – newborns – are protected by the immunity passed down through the microbiome they acquire as they pass through the birth canal, as well as from their mother's breast milk, until their own immune systems develop. For the most part, microbes stay in their inoffensive and usually helpful place because they have neither reason nor opportunity to invade. According to J.V. Neel's study of Brazil's Xavante Indians (*American Journal of Human Genetics,* March 1964), if they do gain a foothold in the old and immune-impaired, the resulting illness cannot spread and is hardly ever fatal. Many aboriginal peoples had no word for or experience of disease until they were subjected to the "civilized" world's modern "medicine."

But even if the germ theory of disease were right, combating infectious disease with vaccines is like holding up your hands to stop the rain. There are millions of microbial varieties and species, and these microbes can mutate much faster than pathogen-hunters can track. Vaccines are species- and variety-specific. Anyone who can do basic math can see how insane the whole enterprise is, even on its own allopathic terms. Both in theory and practice, vaccination is allopathy's superstitious and self-contradictory reduction to absurdity.

Microbes aren't the enemy. Yes, the microbes that stage a frontal assault against the innate immune system trigger a symptomatic response that can be fatal to someone whose immune system has been weakened by hunger, junk food, smoking, drugs, alcohol, overwork, poor sanitation and hygiene, and yes, vaccines. To someone with an exhausted immune system, the common cold or a case of measles can mean death, and no vaccine can prevent that. But in a healthy individual this response, like the spots and fever of measles, is the innate immune system's way of isolating and destroying the invader. Only the microbes that make it into the bloodstream and overwhelm the adaptive immune system trigger the destructive response that we call "disease."

Yet that is exactly what vaccination enables. It suppresses the innate immune system, leaving the individual open to asymptomatic infection that is as contagious as the symptomatic kind but without the benefit of lasting immunity, and also much more dangerous because the infectious agent is enabled to enter the blood stream. And by suppressing the innate immune system, as does most of modern medicine, vaccination can give the impression that it is suppressing disease when in reality it's making things much worse.

The cardinal rule in fighting an epidemic is to minimize and isolate the centers of contagion, but vaccination multiplies those centers by the millions. The cardinal rule of surgery is to maintain a sterile environment to prevent internal infection. Why then does mainstream medicine tout vaccination as one of the greatest medical advances of all time? It takes microbes that would otherwise be benign or easily repelled and injects them into the inner sanctum where they can wreak havoc in all sorts of ways, the worst of which probably are as yet unknown. In doing so, vaccination bypasses the innate immune system and sets up the human organism for attack from within, the kind of attack in all its evolutionary history it has rarely, if ever, had to face. And if it did face such an attack, it was from one "rogue" microbe that made its way through the innate immune system and would be zapped by the forewarned antibodies of the adaptive immune system.

If immunity is the same as organic harmony, vaccination leads to civil war. A vaccine is a biological terrorist, pure and simple. It forces the body into a state of martial law, diverting the energy that otherwise would be used to maintain and improve health toward the formation of antibody SWAT teams that lack any real target and take out their frustration on the very organism they are meant to protect. Autoimmunity, anyone?

Just look at what we do with vaccinations. We inject multiple microbes into infants, and keep on doing so at regular intervals all the way to adulthood and even beyond. Yes, these microbes are "attenuated" or even "inactivated," but a 2008 study published in the *Journal of Virology* [http://jvi.asm.org/content/83/1/117.full] found that an inactivated SV40 virus (the same virus that contaminated the Salk polio vaccine for thirty years and has been deemed even by establishment experts to be highly carcinogenic) can cause DNA damage by its mere presentation. In other words, when it comes to a virus, what you see is what you get. The terrifying appearance is just as harmful as the physiological reality. And those are just the microbes we know about, not the hitchhikers for which testing is not only inadequate but impossible.

Along with the microbes come poisons like aluminum, formaldehyde and mercury that further suppress the innate immune system, clog up and in some cases melt down the nervous system, and enable the microbes to cross the blood-brain barrier where antibodies are too big to follow. There these microbes can mutate unmolested into varieties far more dangerous than their originals because they have learned to commandeer the central nervous system and make it serve their needs, not those of their human host. Meanwhile, the innate immune system is helpless to stop such an enemy in the rear, while the adaptive immune system is so hopelessly confused and overwhelmed that it turns against the organism of which it is an integral part and we get the whole host of auto-immune disorders that are the plague of today's world. And that list is growing as the vaccination schedule does.

In a televised interview with Robert F. Kennedy, Jr., [http://www.boughtmovie.com/robert-f-kennedy-jr-real-time-with-bill-maher/], a crusader against mercury in vaccines, Bill Maher asked why, if vaccines are so bad, are most Americans fairly healthy. Are they really? Nearly half the population suffers from at least one chronic disease, and chronic disease is the leading cause of disability and death [http://www.fightchronicdisease.org/sites/fightchronicdisease.org/files/docs/GrowingCrisisofChronicDiseaseintheUSfactsheet_81009.pdf]. Diseases that were either unknown or confined to the very old before the advent of mass vaccinations are on an astronomical rise in direct statistical correlation with the periodic increases in the vaccination schedule as well as the rise of factory farming, GMOs and glyphosate; widespread use of prescription and over-the-counter drugs; tobacco, alcohol and processed-sugar consumption; a sedentary and sleep-deprived lifestyle; and omnipresent environmental pollution. But vaccination is different from all these other lethal threats for two reasons.

One, vaccination poisons life at the wellspring. What's the point of giving your children healthy food, pure water, and a non-toxic environment, one might wonder, if from the day they're born poison is regularly injected into their veins?

Two, the health establishment as well as most people recognize all those other threats as problems, but they see vaccination as a solution. When it comes to vaccines, the human race is like the proverbial frog in the cooking pot who has the heat raised on him so gradually that before he knows it he's boiled alive.

People like Mark Bittman (also a NY Times columnist) who are against GMOs and chemical pollution but favor vaccination are inconsistent, to put it politely. Vaccine antigens are the original GMOs. Mercury, formaldehyde, aluminum, etc. are harmful in the environment but not when injected into the bloodstream? At least people like George W. Bush and Barack Obama, who proclaim both vaccines and GMOs to be key to a prosperous high-tech future, are consistent. Naive at best and evil at worst, but consistent.

The pharmaceutical corporations, with the active complicity of governments all over the world, are gang-raping the human race. Vaccines are their business plan for the 21st century and it can't be beat: everyone, the healthy as well as the sick, is a potential customer; every little discomfort, like childhood earache and colic, can have a vaccine; unlike with other drugs, in many countries there's no legal liability for the manufacturer; governments subsidize vaccine development and are forcing people to shoot up these pathogenic cocktails; and best of all, people piously thank the vaccination witch-doctors for saving them from the pandemics that can only come through the very vaccines that supposedly will prevent them. The sky's the limit! At least until the market goes extinct.

When this is all so obvious to anyone with eyes to see, why do so many people, even people who are critical of Big Pharma, stop their critical thinking when it comes to vaccines? Why do they trust what the medical, corporate and government mouthpieces say about vaccines even when they mistrust them about everything else?

"It's the economy, stupid." No doubt in large part. The "health-care" industry keeps gobbling up more and more of the GNP pie, so more and more people depend on it for their livelihood. And, of course, money talks. Big Pharma is bigger than Big Oil, bigger than any other corporate mafia in the world. The American Medical Association does its bidding, as do doctors whom the drug reps wine and dine; as do the major media outlets, much of whose advertising revenue comes from Big Pharma; as do research scientists, to whom pharmaceutical companies furnish generous grants as long as those lead to vaccine validation; as do politicians, whom Big Pharma tirelessly lobbies and to whom it gives lavish campaign contributions; as do public health officials all the way up to cabinet level, who have cushy careers awaiting them when they leave the public sector in that epitome of government corruption, the "revolving door" syndrome.

But then why do you often hear criticism of

the medical/pharmaceutical establishment when it comes to other drugs and medical practices, but not, except from the "fringe," when it comes to vaccination?

Vaccination is the quintessence of the religion of the modern world: technology. Not science. Technology. They are not the same thing, but they are so frequently mistaken for each other that technology is in the process of committing identity theft against science with almost no one being the wiser.

The technocrats of the world believe themselves smarter than nature. They are the masters of the universe who will tame nature and, like a trained seal, place her at our beck and call. But so far just about all they've produced is death. Their greatest technological boast is nuclear energy, whose most spectacular manifestation is bombs that can destroy all life on this planet in a matter of minutes. They claim it has peaceful uses like the generation of electricity, but we all know how that's worked out at Three Mile Island and Fukushima.

Then, of course, there are computers and cell phones and all that electronic stuff. But however addicted you may be to your iPhone or game console, you really have to admit that you could survive, and perhaps even have a much more satisfying social life, without them. And the same goes for society as a whole. Modern electronics is creating just as many problems as solutions. It provides tools that are useful but also double-edged.

And mention also has to be made of modern agriculture, with its factory farms and GMOs, as well as the food-processing industry, all of which together are turning our farmland into wasteland, killing off the bees and butterflies without whom so many fruits and vegetables cannot grow, and instead of real food giving us poisonous garbage.

So what's left? Modern medicine, which with its antibiotics and vaccines has allegedly conquered disease and spread goodness and light. But what if it's a gigantic scam, a stupendous hoax? Modern medicine may have a positive role as emergency medicine, but what if in taking over all medicine it's done in human society what vaccines do in the human body – turned every little illness into a medical emergency? What if the drugs that are its staple are killing rather than healing?

Well, then, we'd have to stop blaming demons or microbes and the stars or our genes for our health problems. We'd have to own up to the fact that the fault lies in ourselves, both individually and collectively. We'd have to turn to an alternative medicine that builds on tradition and works with nature and not against it, a truly empirical and scientific medicine that isn't controlled by money-hungry corporate executives and power-hungry politicians. We'd have to eat right, live right, and do right by each other and the environment without which, incidentally, we cannot survive.

There is no moral equivalence between the pro- and anti-vaccine positions. The notorious anti-vaxxers aren't trying to force the opposition to give up its precious vaccines. They just want the freedom not to have the poisons injected into their own veins or the veins of their children. They are confident that, over time, society will wake up from its herd-immunity pipe-dream when it sees how much better off human beings are without vaccines. Indeed, the few studies undertaken by scientists willing to buck the establishment, notably in New Zealand and Germany, show that the unvaccinated are many times healthier than the vaccinated, mentally and emotionally as well as physically. [http://vactruth.com/2014/02/26/unvaccinated-children-healthier/] But the vaccine establishment wants to eliminate all possibility of comparison. In the double-speak through-the-looking-glass logic characteristic of all totalitarian movements, such studies are "unethical."

And make no mistake, the pro-vaccine movement is totalitarian. In the pursuit of a chimerical, biologically impossible vaccine-induced herd immunity, it wants to force everyone to be fully vaccinated. With new vaccines being fast-tracked by the FDA and added by the CDC to the "recommended" schedule every year, as well as new legislation being introduced and passed by state legislatures, the noose is steadily tightening not just on anti-vaxxers but all Americans. With most governments in the world in varying degrees following suit, the right to do everything one can to ensure the health of oneself and one's children is already gone or fast being extinguished.

Whether in pursuit of witches, heretics, Jews, Blacks, or other inconvenient minorities, fear-crazed mobs have always targeted scapegoats at the bidding of their masters. Anti-vaxxers are the new public enemy number one. One way or another, they need to be crushed. This is the ironical real-life context of Frank Bruni's "Vaccine Lunacy."

So, no matter how exalted your professional status, corporate position, or political or judicial office, here's what I say to everyone who, out of hysteria, greed, the will to power, ignorance, self-righteousness or misplaced idealism supports the totalitarian push to shove the vaccination needle into the arm of every human being on the face of the planet:

Vaccines poison life at the wellspring. Shoot up at your own peril.

Compulsory vaccination is assault and battery. Don't commit that crime against my children or me.

Compulsory mass vaccination is slow-motion genocide. Don't commit that crime against the human race.

To answer Dr. Offit's question, would Jesus have made millions and billions of dollars off the repeated injection of multiple pathogens and poisons into the veins of children under the obscene pretext of saving them from disease? Not if he really meant it when he said, "What does it profit a man to gain the whole world and lose his own soul?" (Mark 8:36)

And to those who innocently trust the medical establishment when it comes to vaccines, Jesus also has something apposite to say: "Beware of wolves in sheep's clothing" (Matthew 7:15). Whatever you may think about vaccination at the moment, it's a subject for which there is no excuse, especially for parents, not to study in depth. If you do I warrant you will find, as I did, that all the bluster lies on the side of the pro-vaccination establishment, but all the real science supports the anti-vaxxer "wing-nuts." The absolute moral imperative is to open your mind, do the homework the likes of Paul Offit and Frank Bruni so studiously avoid [A good place to start is Miller's Review of Critical Vaccine Studies: http://www.amazon.com/Millers-Review-Critical-Vaccine-Studies/dp/188121740X/ref=sr_1_1?s=books&ie

=UTF8&qid=1451509899&sr=1-
1&keywords=miller%27s+review+of+critical+v
accine+studies], and then do anything and
everything you can to stop this gradual but
wholesale slaughter of the innocents.

www.ingramcontent.com/pod-product-compliance
Lightning Source LLC
Chambersburg PA
CBHW051134250726

48655CB00007B/3051